Netter's Atlas of the Urinary System in Overactive Bladder

**Illustrations by
Frank H. Netter, M.D.**

Compliments of Novartis Pharmaceuticals Corporation

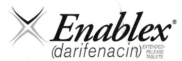
Enablex®
(darifenacin) EXTENDED-RELEASE TABLETS

Icon Custom Communications · Carlstadt, New Jersey

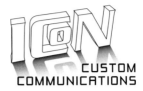

NOTICE

Printed in U.S.A.

Frank Netter: The Physician, The Artist, The Art

This selection of the art of Dr. Frank H. Netter on neuroanatomy and neurophysiology is drawn from *Netter's Atlas of Human Physiology*. Viewing these pictures again prompts reflection on Dr. Netter's work and his roles as physician and artist.

Frank H. Netter was born in 1906 in New York City. He pursued his artistic muse at the Sorbonne, the Art Student's League, and the National Academy of Design before entering medical school at New York University, where he received his M.D. degree in 1931. During his student years, Dr. Netter's notebook sketches attracted the attention of the medical faculty and other physicians, allowing him to augment his income by illustrating articles and textbooks. He continued illustrating as a sideline after establishing a surgical practice in 1933, but ultimately opted to give up his practice in favor of a full-time commitment to art. After service in the United States Army during the Second World War, Dr. Netter began his long collaboration with the CIBA Pharmaceutical Company (now Novartis Pharmaceuticals). This 45-year partnership resulted in the production of the extraordinary collection of medical art so familiar to physicians and other medical professionals worldwide.

When Dr. Netter's work is discussed, attention is focused primarily on Netter the artist and only secondarily on Netter the physician. As a student of Dr. Netter's work for more than forty years, I can say that the true strength of a Netter illustration was always established well before brush was laid to paper. In that respect each plate is more of an intellectual than an artistic or aesthetic exercise. It is easy to appreciate the aesthetic qualities of Dr. Netter's work, but to overlook its intellectual qualities is to miss the real strength and intent of the art. This intellectual process requires thorough understanding of the topic, as Dr. Netter wrote: "Strange as it may seem, the hardest part of making a medical picture is not the drawing at all. It is the planning, the conception, the determination of point of view and the approach which will best clarify the subject which takes the most effort."

Years before the inception of "the integrated curriculum," Netter the physician realized that a good medical illustration can include clinical information and physiologic functions as well as anatomy. In pursuit of this principle, Dr. Netter often integrates pertinent basic and clinical science elements in his anatomic interpretations. Although he was chided for this heresy by a prominent European anatomy professor, many generations of students training to be physicians rather than anatomists have appreciated Dr. Netter's concept.

The integration of physiology and clinical medicine with anatomy has led Dr. Netter to another, more subtle, choice in his art. Many texts and atlases published during the period of Dr. Netter's career depict anatomy clearly based on cadaver specimens with renderings of shrunken and shriveled tissues and organs. Netter the physician chose to render "live" versions of these structures—not shriveled, colorless, formaldehyde-soaked tissues, but plump, robust organs, glowing with color!

The value of Dr. Netter's approach is clearly demonstrated by the plates in this selection.

John A. Craig, M.D.
Austin, Texas

Table of Contents

Anatomy of the Urinary System

Physiology of the Urinary System

Overactive Bladder

Muscarinic Receptors

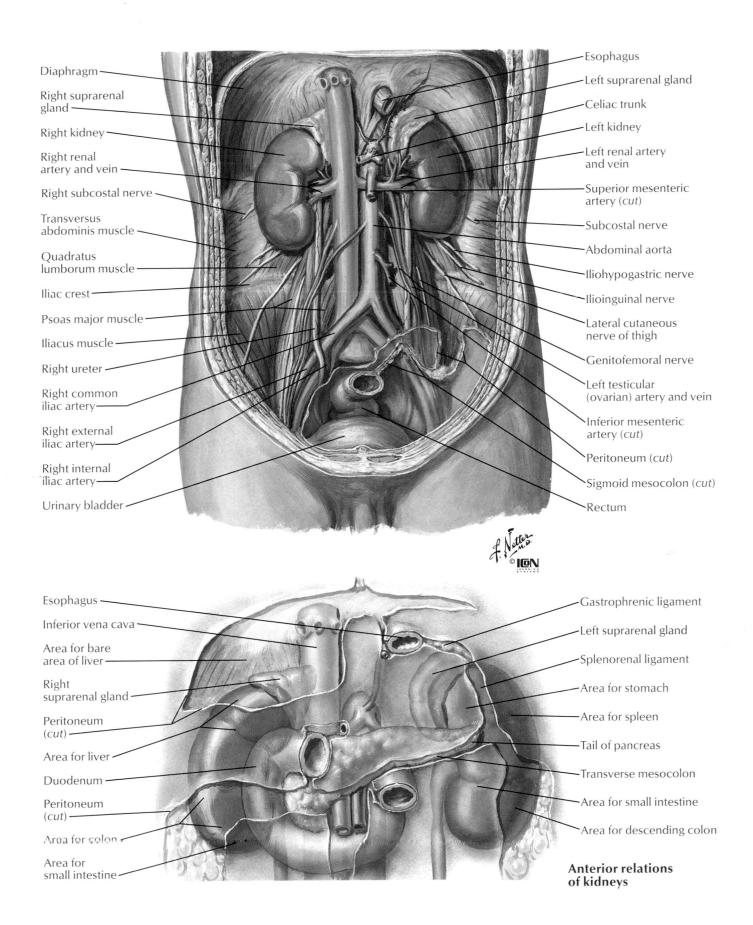

Diaphragm

Right suprarenal gland

Right kidney

Right renal artery and vein

Right subcostal nerve

Transversus abdominis muscle

Quadratus lumborum muscle

Iliac crest

Psoas major muscle

Iliacus muscle

Right ureter

Right common iliac artery

Right external iliac artery

Right internal iliac artery

Urinary bladder

Esophagus

Left suprarenal gland

Celiac trunk

Left kidney

Left renal artery and vein

Superior mesenteric artery (*cut*)

Subcostal nerve

Abdominal aorta

Iliohypogastric nerve

Ilioinguinal nerve

Lateral cutaneous nerve of thigh

Genitofemoral nerve

Left testicular (ovarian) artery and vein

Inferior mesenteric artery (*cut*)

Peritoneum (*cut*)

Sigmoid mesocolon (*cut*)

Rectum

Esophagus

Inferior vena cava

Area for bare area of liver

Right suprarenal gland

Peritoneum (*cut*)

Area for liver

Duodenum

Peritoneum (*cut*)

Area for colon

Area for small intestine

Gastrophrenic ligament

Left suprarenal gland

Splenorenal ligament

Area for stomach

Area for spleen

Tail of pancreas

Transverse mesocolon

Area for small intestine

Area for descending colon

Anterior relations of kidneys

1

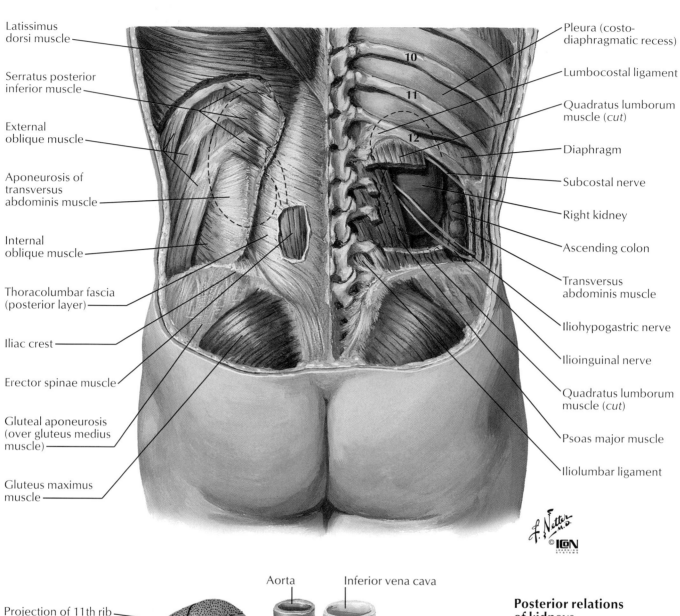

Latissimus dorsi muscle

Serratus posterior inferior muscle

External oblique muscle

Aponeurosis of transversus abdominis muscle

Internal oblique muscle

Thoracolumbar fascia (posterior layer)

Iliac crest

Erector spinae muscle

Gluteal aponeurosis (over gluteus medius muscle)

Gluteus maximus muscle

Pleura (costo-diaphragmatic recess)

Lumbocostal ligament

Quadratus lumborum muscle (cut)

Diaphragm

Subcostal nerve

Right kidney

Ascending colon

Transversus abdominis muscle

Iliohypogastric nerve

Ilioinguinal nerve

Quadratus lumborum muscle (cut)

Psoas major muscle

Iliolumbar ligament

10
11
12

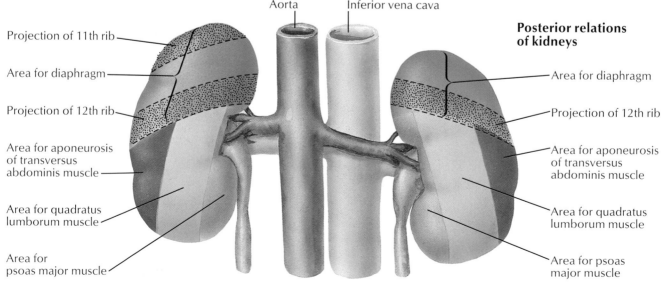

Aorta   Inferior vena cava

Posterior relations of kidneys

Projection of 11th rib

Area for diaphragm

Projection of 12th rib

Area for aponeurosis of transversus abdominis muscle

Area for quadratus lumborum muscle

Area for psoas major muscle

Area for diaphragm

Projection of 12th rib

Area for aponeurosis of transversus abdominis muscle

Area for quadratus lumborum muscle

Area for psoas major muscle

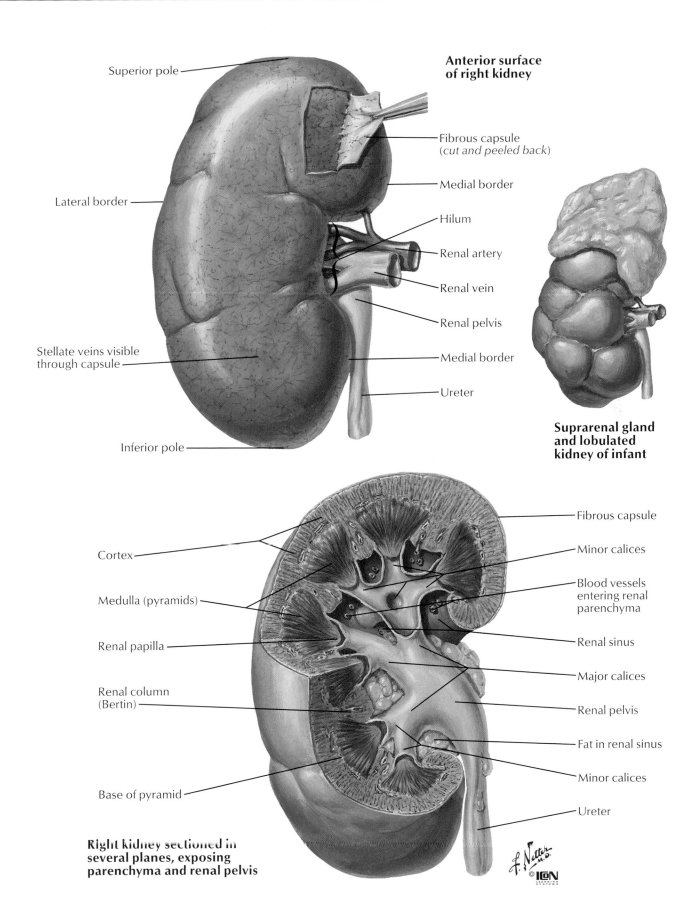

Superior pole

Anterior surface of right kidney

Fibrous capsule (*cut and peeled back*)

Medial border

Hilum

Renal artery

Lateral border

Renal vein

Renal pelvis

Stellate veins visible through capsule

Medial border

Ureter

Inferior pole

Suprarenal gland and lobulated kidney of infant

Cortex

Fibrous capsule

Minor calices

Medulla (pyramids)

Blood vessels entering renal parenchyma

Renal papilla

Renal sinus

Major calices

Renal column (Bertin)

Renal pelvis

Fat in renal sinus

Minor calices

Base of pyramid

Ureter

Right kidney sectioned in several planes, exposing parenchyma and renal pelvis

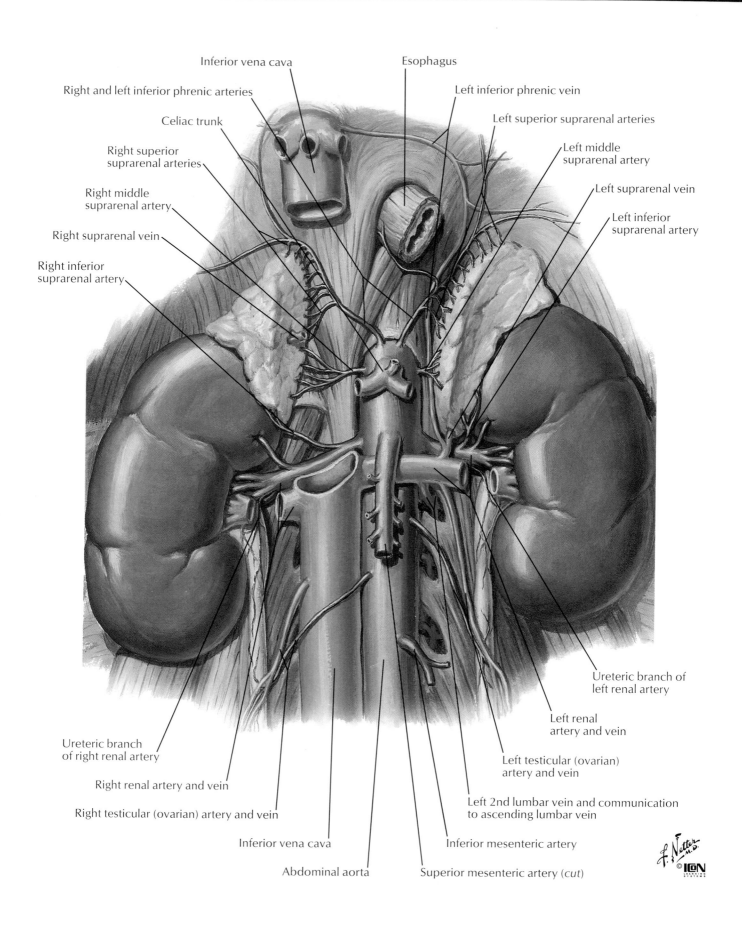

Inferior vena cava

Esophagus

Right and left inferior phrenic arteries

Left inferior phrenic vein

Celiac trunk

Left superior suprarenal arteries

Right superior suprarenal arteries

Left middle suprarenal artery

Right middle suprarenal artery

Left suprarenal vein

Right suprarenal vein

Left inferior suprarenal artery

Right inferior suprarenal artery

Ureteric branch of left renal artery

Left renal artery and vein

Ureteric branch of right renal artery

Left testicular (ovarian) artery and vein

Right renal artery and vein

Left 2nd lumbar vein and communication to ascending lumbar vein

Right testicular (ovarian) artery and vein

Inferior vena cava

Inferior mesenteric artery

Abdominal aorta

Superior mesenteric artery (cut)

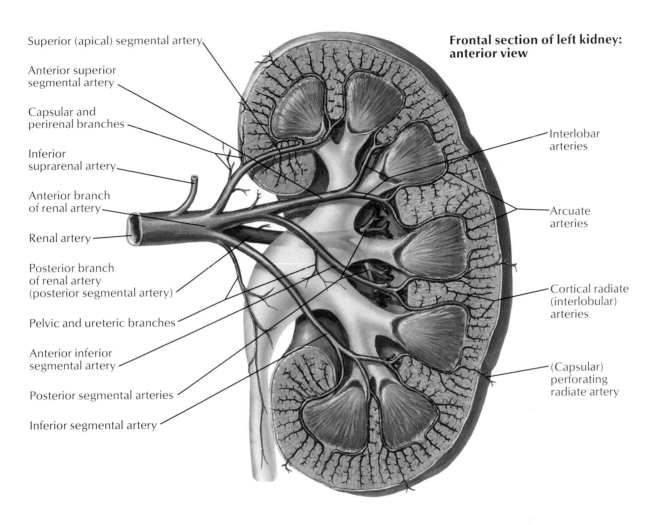

Superior (apical) segmental artery

Anterior superior segmental artery

Capsular and perirenal branches

Inferior suprarenal artery

Anterior branch of renal artery

Renal artery

Posterior branch of renal artery (posterior segmental artery)

Pelvic and ureteric branches

Anterior inferior segmental artery

Posterior segmental arteries

Inferior segmental artery

Frontal section of left kidney: anterior view

Interlobar arteries

Arcuate arteries

Cortical radiate (interlobular) arteries

(Capsular) perforating radiate artery

Vascular renal segments

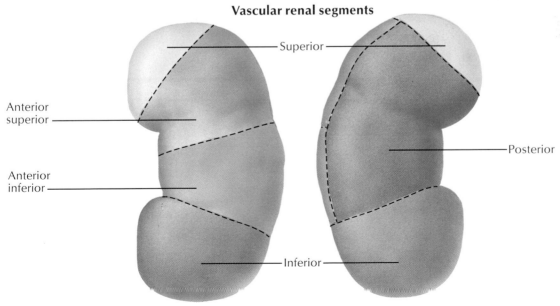

Superior

Anterior superior

Anterior inferior

Posterior

Inferior

Anterior surface of left kidney

Posterior surface of left kidney

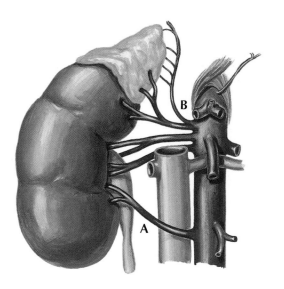

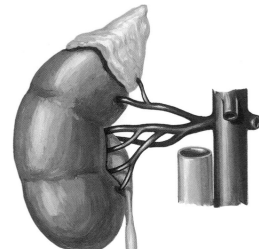

Proximal
subdivision
of renal
artery

A Low accessory right renal
artery may pass anterior to inferior
vena cava instead of posterior to it

B Inferior phrenic artery with
superior suprarenal arteries may arise
from renal artery (middle suprarenal
artery absent)

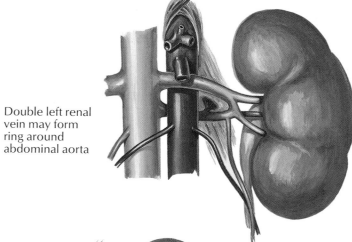

Double left renal
vein may form
ring around
abdominal aorta

Multiple renal veins

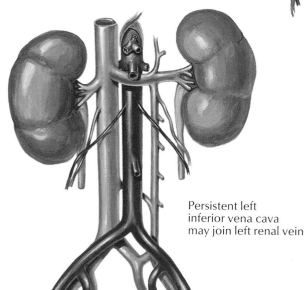

Persistent left
inferior vena cava
may join left renal vein

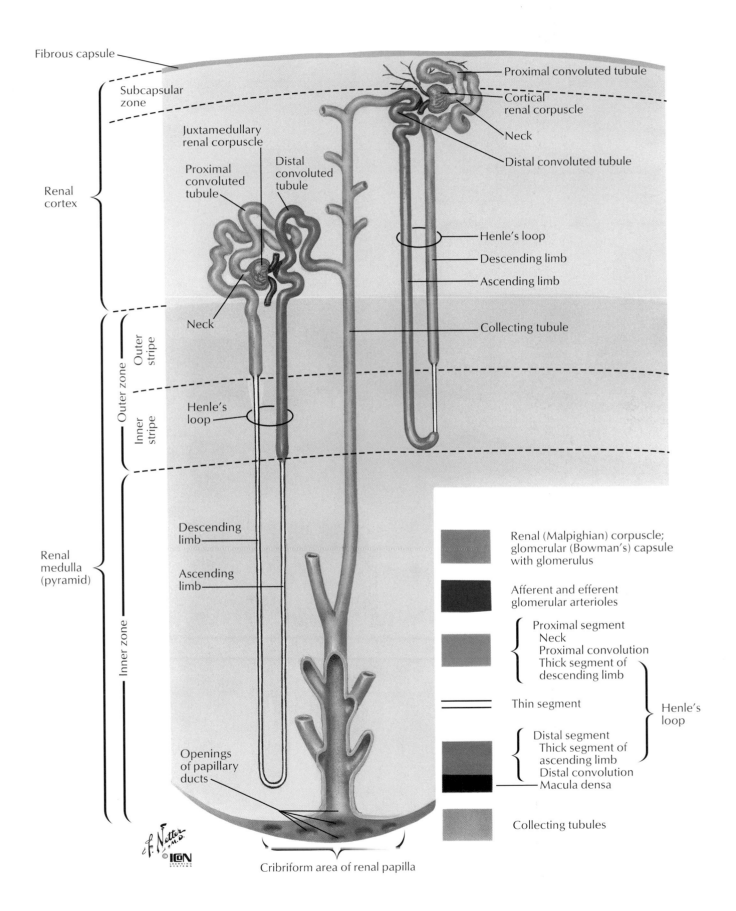

Fibrous capsule

Subcapsular zone

Renal cortex

Juxtamedullary renal corpuscle

Proximal convoluted tubule

Distal convoluted tubule

Neck

Proximal convoluted tubule

Cortical renal corpuscle

Neck

Distal convoluted tubule

Henle's loop

Descending limb

Ascending limb

Collecting tubule

Outer zone

Outer stripe

Inner stripe

Henle's loop

Renal medulla (pyramid)

Inner zone

Descending limb

Ascending limb

Openings of papillary ducts

Cribriform area of renal papilla

Renal (Malpighian) corpuscle; glomerular (Bowman's) capsule with glomerulus

Afferent and efferent glomerular arterioles

Proximal segment
Neck
Proximal convolution
Thick segment of descending limb

Thin segment

Henle's loop

Distal segment
Thick segment of ascending limb
Distal convolution
Macula densa

Collecting tubules

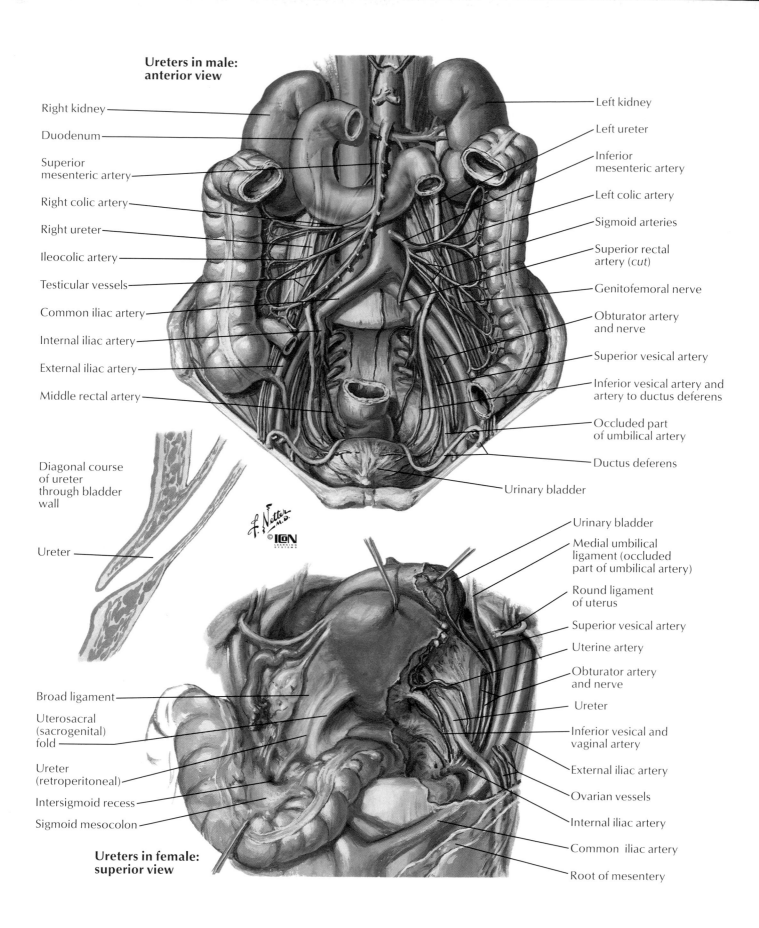

Ureters in male: anterior view

Right kidney

Duodenum

Superior mesenteric artery

Right colic artery

Right ureter

Ileocolic artery

Testicular vessels

Common iliac artery

Internal iliac artery

External iliac artery

Middle rectal artery

Left kidney

Left ureter

Inferior mesenteric artery

Left colic artery

Sigmoid arteries

Superior rectal artery (cut)

Genitofemoral nerve

Obturator artery and nerve

Superior vesical artery

Inferior vesical artery and artery to ductus deferens

Occluded part of umbilical artery

Ductus deferens

Urinary bladder

Diagonal course of ureter through bladder wall

Ureter

Broad ligament

Uterosacral (sacrogenital) fold

Ureter (retroperitoneal)

Intersigmoid recess

Sigmoid mesocolon

Ureters in female: superior view

Urinary bladder

Medial umbilical ligament (occluded part of umbilical artery)

Round ligament of uterus

Superior vesical artery

Uterine artery

Obturator artery and nerve

Ureter

Inferior vesical and vaginal artery

External iliac artery

Ovarian vessels

Internal iliac artery

Common iliac artery

Root of mesentery

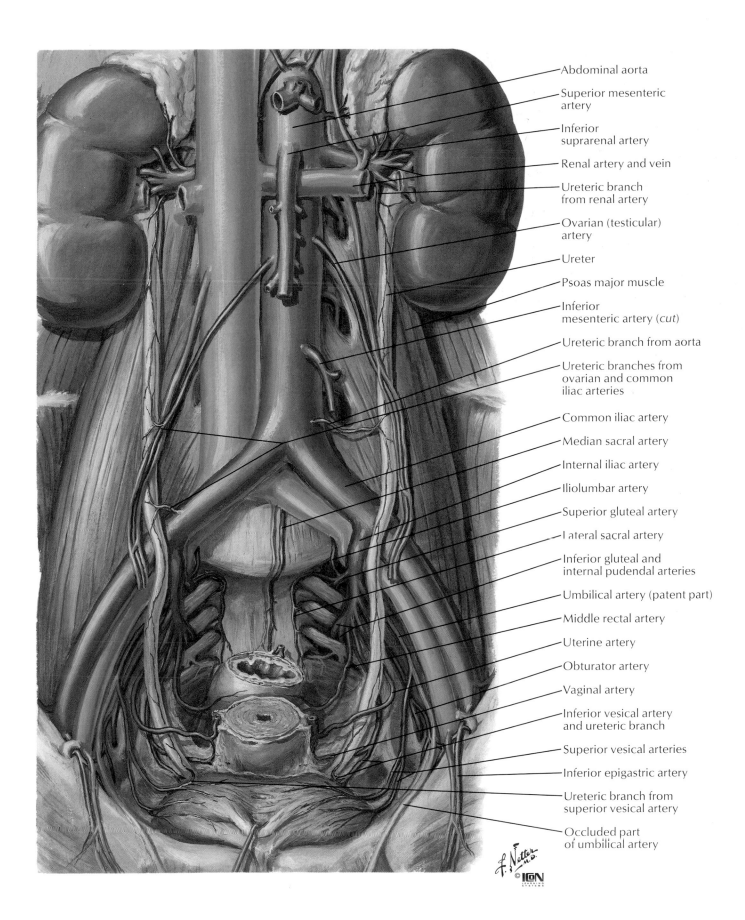

Abdominal aorta

Superior mesenteric artery

Inferior suprarenal artery

Renal artery and vein

Ureteric branch from renal artery

Ovarian (testicular) artery

Ureter

Psoas major muscle

Inferior mesenteric artery (*cut*)

Ureteric branch from aorta

Ureteric branches from ovarian and common iliac arteries

Common iliac artery

Median sacral artery

Internal iliac artery

Iliolumbar artery

Superior gluteal artery

Lateral sacral artery

Inferior gluteal and internal pudendal arteries

Umbilical artery (patent part)

Middle rectal artery

Uterine artery

Obturator artery

Vaginal artery

Inferior vesical artery and ureteric branch

Superior vesical arteries

Inferior epigastric artery

Ureteric branch from superior vesical artery

Occluded part of umbilical artery

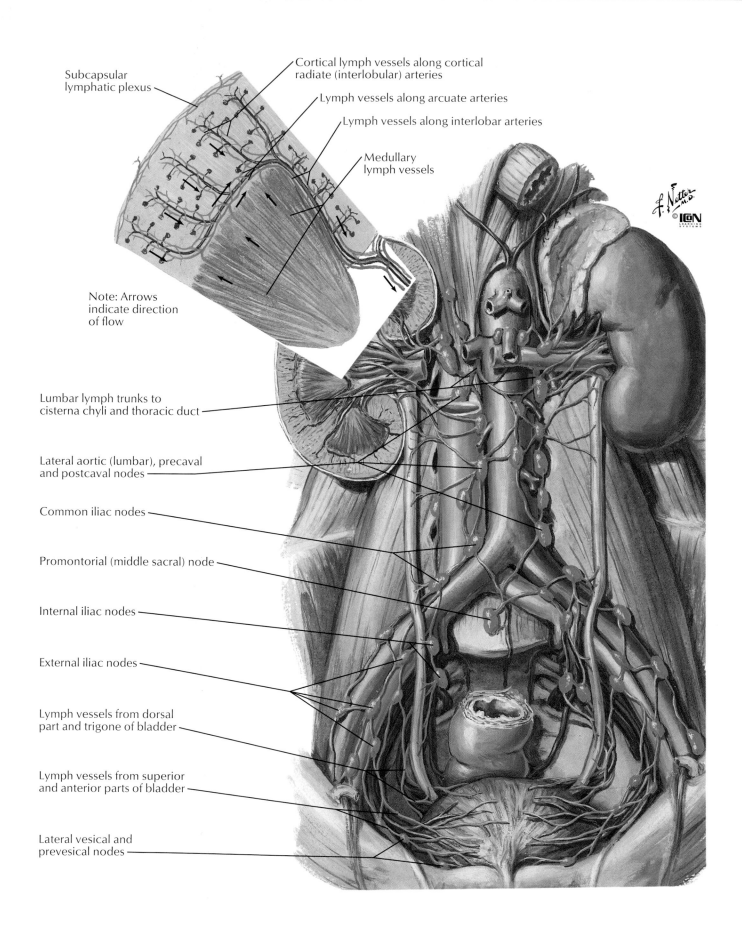

Subcapsular lymphatic plexus

Cortical lymph vessels along cortical radiate (interlobular) arteries

Lymph vessels along arcuate arteries

Lymph vessels along interlobar arteries

Medullary lymph vessels

Note: Arrows indicate direction of flow

Lumbar lymph trunks to cisterna chyli and thoracic duct

Lateral aortic (lumbar), precaval and postcaval nodes

Common iliac nodes

Promontorial (middle sacral) node

Internal iliac nodes

External iliac nodes

Lymph vessels from dorsal part and trigone of bladder

Lymph vessels from superior and anterior parts of bladder

Lateral vesical and prevesical nodes

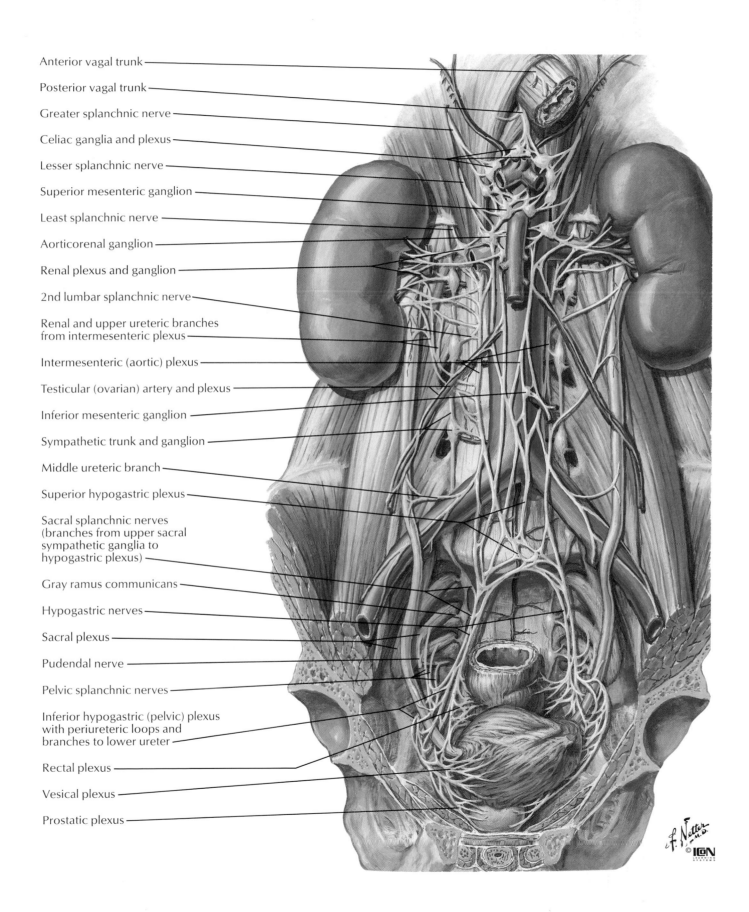

Anterior vagal trunk

Posterior vagal trunk

Greater splanchnic nerve

Celiac ganglia and plexus

Lesser splanchnic nerve

Superior mesenteric ganglion

Least splanchnic nerve

Aorticorenal ganglion

Renal plexus and ganglion

2nd lumbar splanchnic nerve

Renal and upper ureteric branches from intermesenteric plexus

Intermesenteric (aortic) plexus

Testicular (ovarian) artery and plexus

Inferior mesenteric ganglion

Sympathetic trunk and ganglion

Middle ureteric branch

Superior hypogastric plexus

Sacral splanchnic nerves (branches from upper sacral sympathetic ganglia to hypogastric plexus)

Gray ramus communicans

Hypogastric nerves

Sacral plexus

Pudendal nerve

Pelvic splanchnic nerves

Inferior hypogastric (pelvic) plexus with periureteric loops and branches to lower ureter

Rectal plexus

Vesical plexus

Prostatic plexus

11

Median (sagittal) section

Sacral promontory

Ureter

Suspensory ligament of ovary

Uterine (Fallopian) tube

Ovary

External iliac vessels

Ligament of ovary

Body of uterus

Round ligament of uterus (ligamentum teres)

Fundus of uterus

Urinary bladder

Pubic symphysis

Urethra

Deep transverse perineal muscle

Inferior (arcuate) pubic ligament

Deep dorsal vein of clitoris

Crus of clitoris

External urethral orifice

Labium minus

Labium majus

Uterosacral ligament

Vesicouterine pouch

Rectouterine pouch (cul-de-sac of Douglas)

Cervix of uterus

Posterior part of vaginal fornix

Anterior part of vaginal fornix

Rectum

Vagina

Levator ani muscle

Anal canal

External anal sphincter muscle

Anus

Vaginal orifice

Paramedian (sagittal) dissection

Ureter

Uterine (Fallopian) tube

Ovary

Ligament of ovary

Round ligament of uterus

Broad ligament (cut)

Superior pubic ramus (cut)

Inferior pubic ramus (cut)

Ischiocavernosus muscle

Body of clitoris

Labia minora

Labium majus

Rectouterine pouch (cul-de-sac of Douglas)

Peritoneum (cut edge)

Vesicouterine pouch

Rectum

Ureter

Urinary bladder

Vagina

Pelvic diaphragm (levator ani muscle)

Deep transverse perineal muscle (cut)

External anal sphincter muscle

12

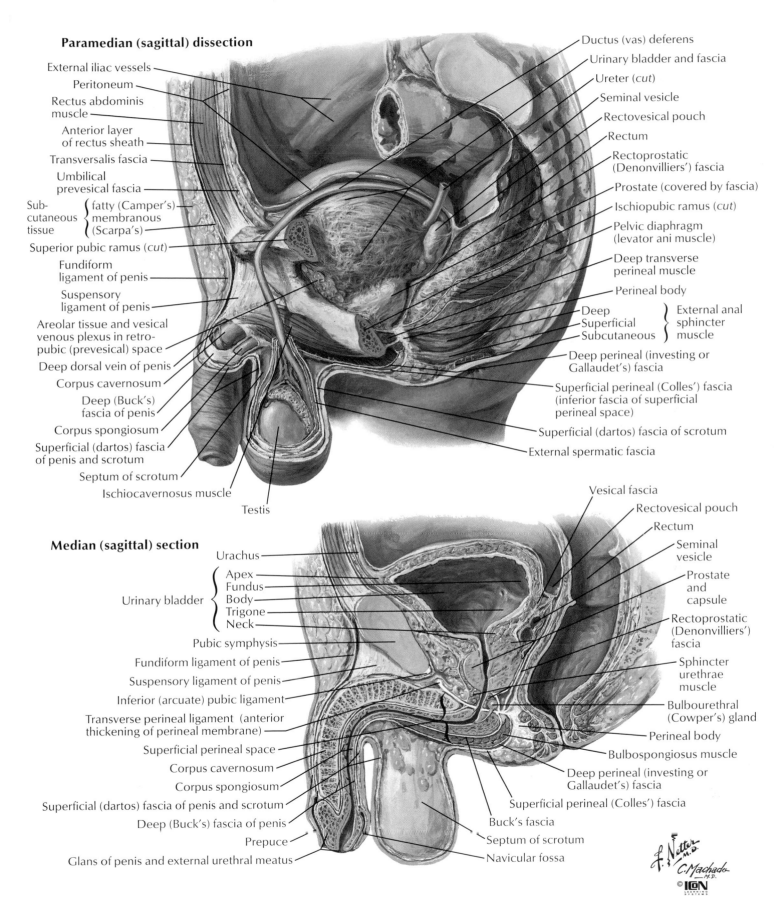

Paramedian (sagittal) dissection

- External iliac vessels
- Peritoneum
- Rectus abdominis muscle
- Anterior layer of rectus sheath
- Transversalis fascia
- Umbilical prevesical fascia
- Sub-cutaneous tissue { fatty (Camper's) / membranous (Scarpa's) }
- Superior pubic ramus (cut)
- Fundiform ligament of penis
- Suspensory ligament of penis
- Areolar tissue and vesical venous plexus in retro-pubic (prevesical) space
- Deep dorsal vein of penis
- Corpus cavernosum
- Deep (Buck's) fascia of penis
- Corpus spongiosum
- Superficial (dartos) fascia of penis and scrotum
- Septum of scrotum
- Ischiocavernosus muscle
- Testis

- Ductus (vas) deferens
- Urinary bladder and fascia
- Ureter (cut)
- Seminal vesicle
- Rectovesical pouch
- Rectum
- Rectoprostatic (Denonvilliers') fascia
- Prostate (covered by fascia)
- Ischiopubic ramus (cut)
- Pelvic diaphragm (levator ani muscle)
- Deep transverse perineal muscle
- Perineal body
- Deep / Superficial / Subcutaneous } External anal sphincter muscle
- Deep perineal (investing or Gallaudet's) fascia
- Superficial perineal (Colles') fascia (inferior fascia of superficial perineal space)
- Superficial (dartos) fascia of scrotum
- External spermatic fascia

Median (sagittal) section

- Urachus
- Urinary bladder { Apex / Fundus / Body / Trigone / Neck }
- Pubic symphysis
- Fundiform ligament of penis
- Suspensory ligament of penis
- Inferior (arcuate) pubic ligament
- Transverse perineal ligament (anterior thickening of perineal membrane)
- Superficial perineal space
- Corpus cavernosum
- Corpus spongiosum
- Superficial (dartos) fascia of penis and scrotum
- Deep (Buck's) fascia of penis
- Prepuce
- Glans of penis and external urethral meatus

- Vesical fascia
- Rectovesical pouch
- Rectum
- Seminal vesicle
- Prostate and capsule
- Rectoprostatic (Denonvilliers') fascia
- Sphincter urethrae muscle
- Bulbourethral (Cowper's) gland
- Perineal body
- Bulbospongiosus muscle
- Deep perineal (investing or Gallaudet's) fascia
- Superficial perineal (Colles') fascia
- Buck's fascia
- Septum of scrotum
- Navicular fossa

F. Netter M.D.
C. Machado M.D.
©ICON LEARNING SYSTEMS

Female: midsagittal section

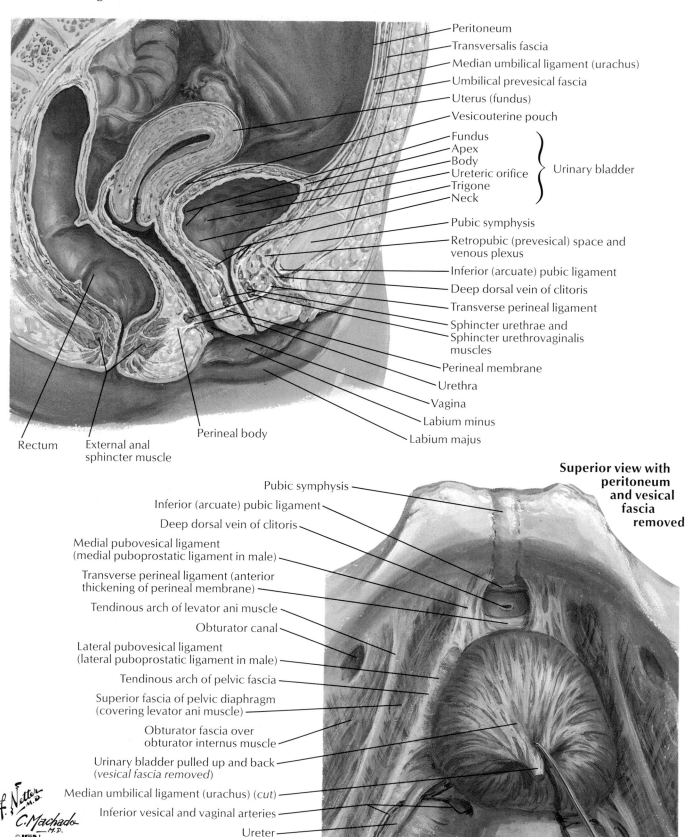

Peritoneum

Transversalis fascia

Median umbilical ligament (urachus)

Umbilical prevesical fascia

Uterus (fundus)

Vesicouterine pouch

Fundus
Apex
Body
Ureteric orifice
Trigone
Neck

Urinary bladder

Pubic symphysis

Retropubic (prevesical) space and venous plexus

Inferior (arcuate) pubic ligament

Deep dorsal vein of clitoris

Transverse perineal ligament

Sphincter urethrae and Sphincter urethrovaginalis muscles

Perineal membrane

Urethra

Vagina

Labium minus

Labium majus

Perineal body

Rectum

External anal sphincter muscle

Superior view with peritoneum and vesical fascia removed

Pubic symphysis

Inferior (arcuate) pubic ligament

Deep dorsal vein of clitoris

Medial pubovesical ligament (medial puboprostatic ligament in male)

Transverse perineal ligament (anterior thickening of perineal membrane)

Tendinous arch of levator ani muscle

Obturator canal

Lateral pubovesical ligament (lateral puboprostatic ligament in male)

Tendinous arch of pelvic fascia

Superior fascia of pelvic diaphragm (covering levator ani muscle)

Obturator fascia over obturator internus muscle

Urinary bladder pulled up and back (*vesical fascia removed*)

Median umbilical ligament (urachus) (*cut*)

Inferior vesical and vaginal arteries

Ureter

14

Female: frontal section

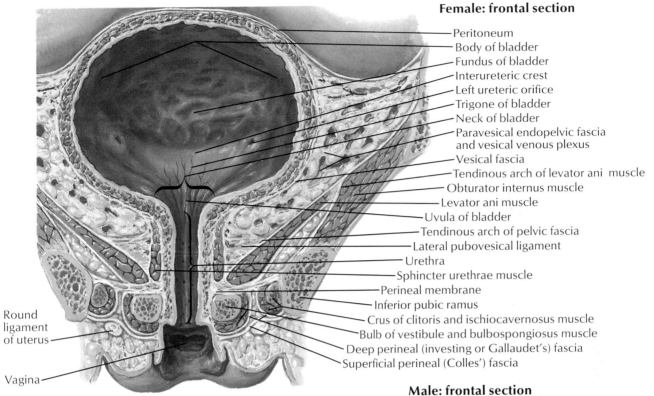

Peritoneum
Body of bladder
Fundus of bladder
Interureteric crest
Left ureteric orifice
Trigone of bladder
Neck of bladder
Paravesical endopelvic fascia and vesical venous plexus
Vesical fascia
Tendinous arch of levator ani muscle
Obturator internus muscle
Levator ani muscle
Uvula of bladder
Tendinous arch of pelvic fascia
Lateral pubovesical ligament
Urethra
Sphincter urethrae muscle
Perineal membrane
Inferior pubic ramus
Crus of clitoris and ischiocavernosus muscle
Bulb of vestibule and bulbospongiosus muscle
Deep perineal (investing or Gallaudet's) fascia
Superficial perineal (Colles') fascia

Round ligament of uterus

Vagina

Male: frontal section

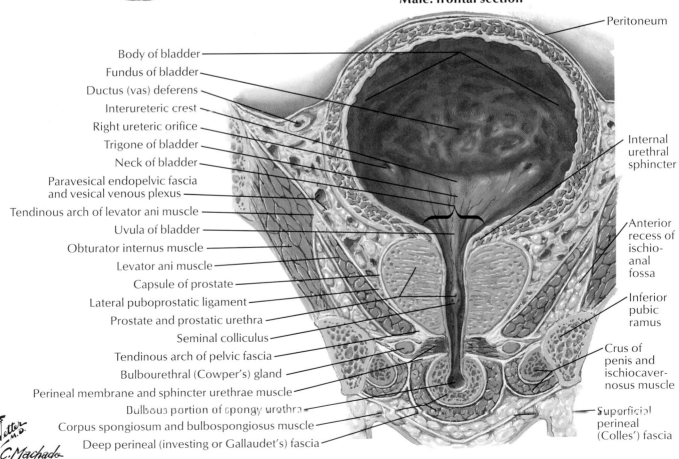

Body of bladder
Fundus of bladder
Ductus (vas) deferens
Interureteric crest
Right ureteric orifice
Trigone of bladder
Neck of bladder
Paravesical endopelvic fascia and vesical venous plexus
Tendinous arch of levator ani muscle
Uvula of bladder
Obturator internus muscle
Levator ani muscle
Capsule of prostate
Lateral puboprostatic ligament
Prostate and prostatic urethra
Seminal colliculus
Tendinous arch of pelvic fascia
Bulbourethral (Cowper's) gland
Perineal membrane and sphincter urethrae muscle
Bulbous portion of spongy urethra
Corpus spongiosum and bulbospongiosus muscle
Deep perineal (investing or Gallaudet's) fascia

Peritoneum

Internal urethral sphincter

Anterior recess of ischio-anal fossa

Inferior pubic ramus

Crus of penis and ischiocavernosus muscle

Superficial perineal (Colles') fascia

F. Netter M.D.
C. Machado M.D.
© ICON LEARNING SYSTEMS

Superior view with peritoneum intact

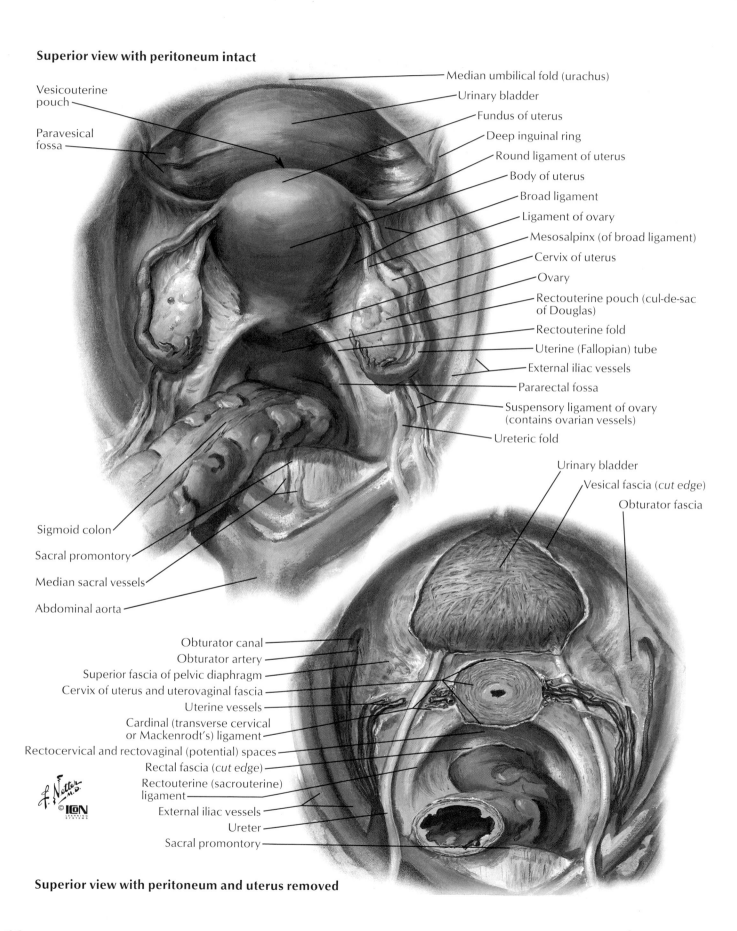

Vesicouterine pouch

Paravesical fossa

Median umbilical fold (urachus)

Urinary bladder

Fundus of uterus

Deep inguinal ring

Round ligament of uterus

Body of uterus

Broad ligament

Ligament of ovary

Mesosalpinx (of broad ligament)

Cervix of uterus

Ovary

Rectouterine pouch (cul-de-sac of Douglas)

Rectouterine fold

Uterine (Fallopian) tube

External iliac vessels

Pararectal fossa

Suspensory ligament of ovary (contains ovarian vessels)

Ureteric fold

Sigmoid colon

Sacral promontory

Median sacral vessels

Abdominal aorta

Urinary bladder

Vesical fascia (*cut edge*)

Obturator fascia

Obturator canal

Obturator artery

Superior fascia of pelvic diaphragm

Cervix of uterus and uterovaginal fascia

Uterine vessels

Cardinal (transverse cervical or Mackenrodt's) ligament

Rectocervical and rectovaginal (potential) spaces

Rectal fascia (*cut edge*)

Rectouterine (sacrouterine) ligament

External iliac vessels

Ureter

Sacral promontory

Superior view with peritoneum and uterus removed

Neurogenic Disorders of the Urinary Bladder

Etiology

Spinal cord

Syphilis
(Tabes dorsalis)
Pernicious anemia
(Subacute com-
bined sclerosis)
Tumors
Trauma
(Transection)
Hematoma
Syringomyelia
Multiple sclerosis
Arteriosclerosis
Poliomyelitis
Transverse myelitis
Paralysis agitans
Disc herniation

L1

L2

Sympathetic
trunk

Key
Sympathetics
Parasympathetics
Sensory
Somatic

Aortic
(inter-
mesenteric)
plexus

S2

S3

S4

Cauda Equina

Tumors
Trauma
Spina Bifida

Cauda
equina

Hypo-
gastric
nerves

Spastic
(Christmas
tree)
bladder
with
sacculation

**Nerves and/or
nerve plexuses**

Trauma
Accidental
Surgical
Diabetes
Neuropathy
Infections
Scarlet fever,
etc.
External pressure
Fetal head
Neoplasm

Pelvic
splanchnic
nerves
(nervi
erigentes)

Inferior
hypogastric
and vesical
plexuses

Flaccid, distended,
atonic bladder
with fine
trabeculation

Pudendal nerves

17

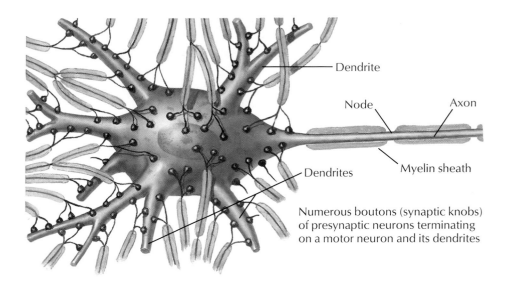

Dendrite

Node

Axon

Myelin sheath

Dendrites

Numerous boutons (synaptic knobs)
of presynaptic neurons terminating
on a motor neuron and its dendrites

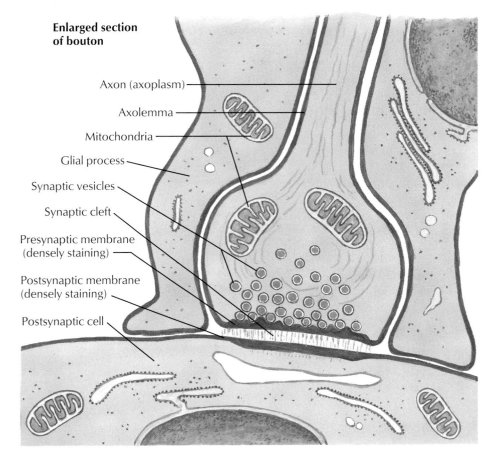

**Enlarged section
of bouton**

Axon (axoplasm)

Axolemma

Mitochondria

Glial process

Synaptic vesicles

Synaptic cleft

Presynaptic membrane
(densely staining)

Postsynaptic membrane
(densely staining)

Postsynaptic cell

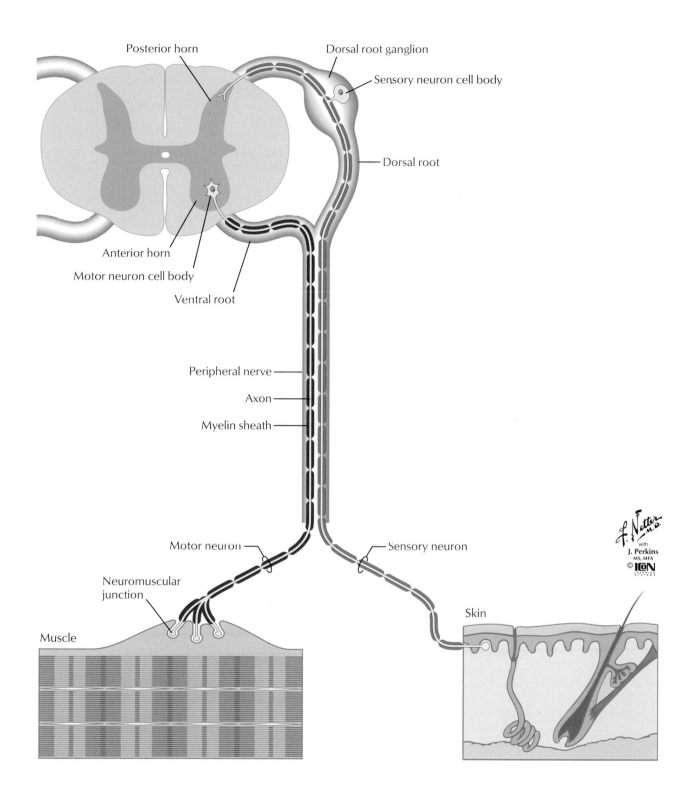

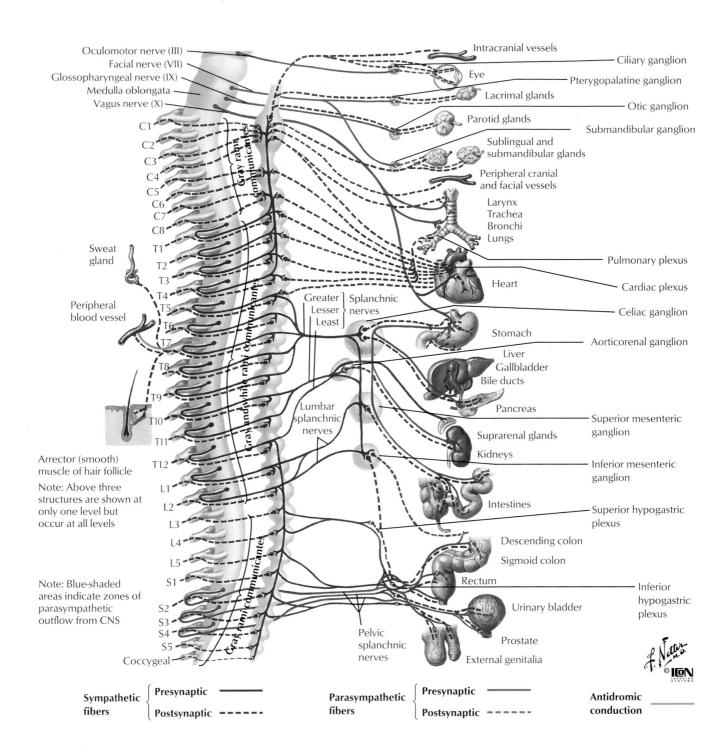

Oculomotor nerve (III)
Facial nerve (VII)
Glossopharyngeal nerve (IX)
Medulla oblongata
Vagus nerve (X)

Intracranial vessels
Ciliary ganglion
Eye
Pterygopalatine ganglion
Lacrimal glands
Otic ganglion
Parotid glands
Submandibular ganglion
Sublingual and submandibular glands
Peripheral cranial and facial vessels
Larynx
Trachea
Bronchi
Lungs
Pulmonary plexus
Heart
Cardiac plexus
Celiac ganglion
Stomach
Aorticorenal ganglion
Liver
Gallbladder
Bile ducts
Pancreas
Superior mesenteric ganglion
Suprarenal glands
Kidneys
Inferior mesenteric ganglion
Intestines
Superior hypogastric plexus
Descending colon
Sigmoid colon
Rectum
Inferior hypogastric plexus
Urinary bladder
Prostate
External genitalia

C1
C2
C3
C4
C5
C6
C7
C8
T1
T2
T3
T4
T5
T6
T7
T8
T9
T10
T11
T12
L1
L2
L3
L4
L5
S1
S2
S3
S4
S5
Coccygeal

Gray rami communicantes

Gray and white rami communicantes

Gray rami communicantes

Greater
Lesser
Least
Splanchnic nerves

Lumbar splanchnic nerves

Pelvic splanchnic nerves

Sweat gland

Peripheral blood vessel

Arrector (smooth) muscle of hair follicle

Note: Above three structures are shown at only one level but occur at all levels

Note: Blue-shaded areas indicate zones of parasympathetic outflow from CNS

| Sympathetic fibers | Presynaptic | —— |
| | Postsynaptic | ------ |

| Parasympathetic fibers | Presynaptic | —— |
| | Postsynaptic | ------ |

Antidromic conduction ——

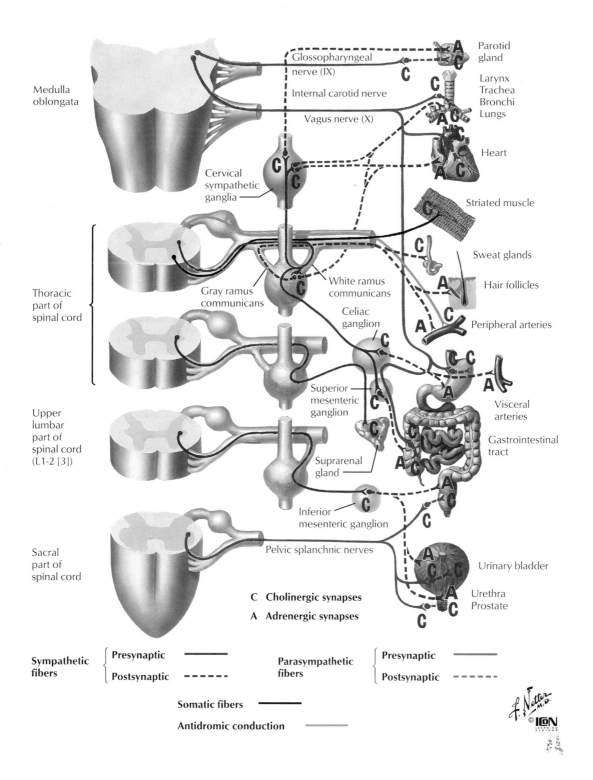

Medulla
oblongata

Glossopharyngeal
nerve (IX)

Internal carotid nerve

Vagus nerve (X)

Parotid
gland

Larynx
Trachea
Bronchi
Lungs

Heart

Cervical
sympathetic
ganglia

Thoracic
part of
spinal cord

Gray ramus
communicans

White ramus
communicans

Celiac
ganglion

Striated muscle

Sweat glands

Hair follicles

Peripheral arteries

Superior
mesenteric
ganglion

Visceral
arteries

Upper
lumbar
part of
spinal cord
(L1-2 [3])

Suprarenal
gland

Gastrointestinal
tract

Inferior
mesenteric ganglion

Sacral
part of
spinal cord

Pelvic splanchnic nerves

Urinary bladder

Urethra
Prostate

C **Cholinergic synapses**

A **Adrenergic synapses**

**Sympathetic
fibers** ⎰ Presynaptic ——————
⎱ Postsynaptic - - - - - -

**Parasympathetic
fibers** ⎰ Presynaptic ——————
⎱ Postsynaptic - - - - - -

Somatic fibers ——————

Antidromic conduction ——————

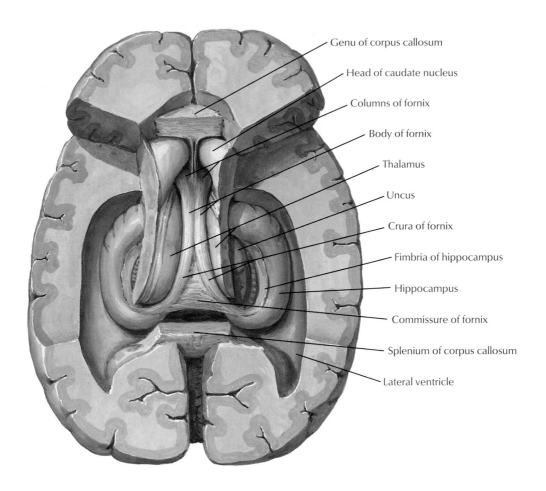

Genu of corpus callosum

Head of caudate nucleus

Columns of fornix

Body of fornix

Thalamus

Uncus

Crura of fornix

Fimbria of hippocampus

Hippocampus

Commissure of fornix

Splenium of corpus callosum

Lateral ventricle

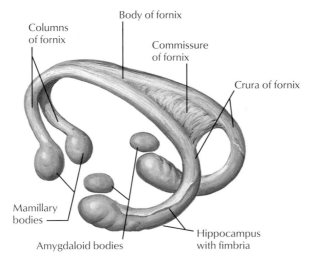

Columns of fornix

Body of fornix

Commissure of fornix

Crura of fornix

Mamillary bodies

Amygdaloid bodies

Hippocampus with fimbria

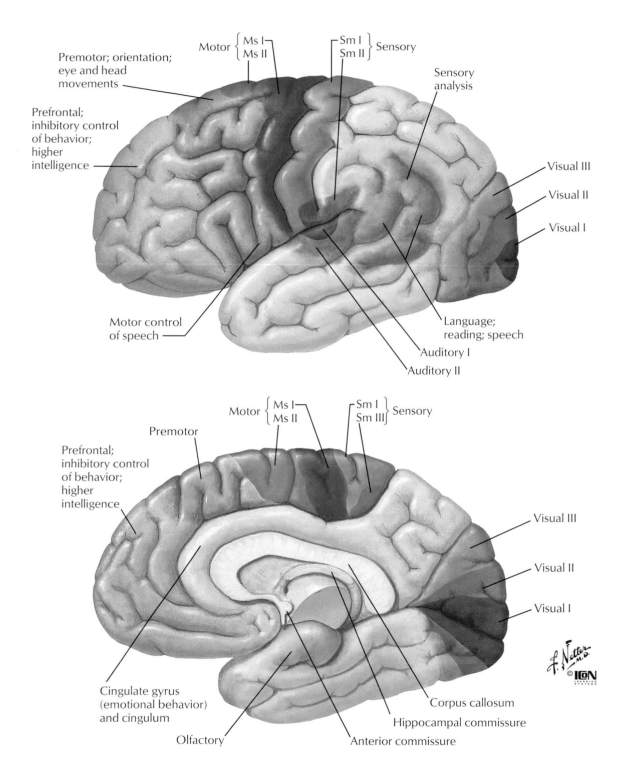

Motor { Ms I — Ms II

Premotor; orientation; eye and head movements

Sm I — Sm II } Sensory

Sensory analysis

Prefrontal; inhibitory control of behavior; higher intelligence

Visual III

Visual II

Visual I

Motor control of speech

Language; reading; speech

Auditory I

Auditory II

Motor { Ms I — Ms II

Premotor

Sm I — Sm III } Sensory

Prefrontal; inhibitory control of behavior; higher intelligence

Visual III

Visual II

Visual I

Cingulate gyrus (emotional behavior) and cingulum

Olfactory

Anterior commissure

Corpus callosum

Hippocampal commissure

J. Perkins
MS, MFA
©ICN
LEARNING
SYSTEMS

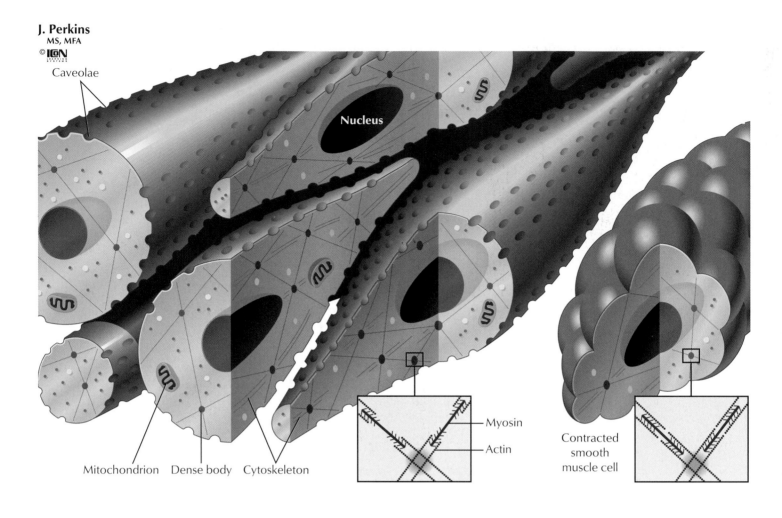

Caveolae

Nucleus

Mitochondrion   Dense body   Cytoskeleton

Myosin

Actin

Contracted
smooth
muscle cell

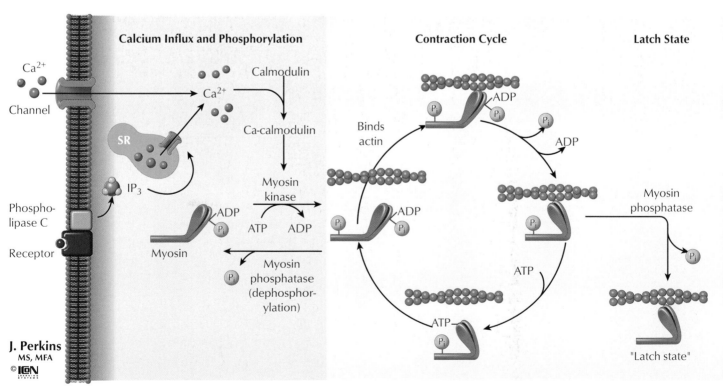

Calcium Influx and Phosphorylation

Contraction Cycle

Latch State

Ca²⁺

Channel

Calmodulin

Ca²⁺

Ca-calmodulin

SR

IP₃

Phospho-
lipase C

Receptor

Myosin

ADP

Pi

ATP   ADP

Myosin
kinase

Myosin
phosphatase
(dephosphor-
ylation)

Pi

Binds
actin

Pi

ADP

Pi

Pi

ADP

Pi

Pi

ADP

Pi

ATP

Pi

ATP

Myosin
phosphatase

Pi

"Latch state"

J. Perkins
MS, MFA
©ICN
LEARNING
SYSTEMS

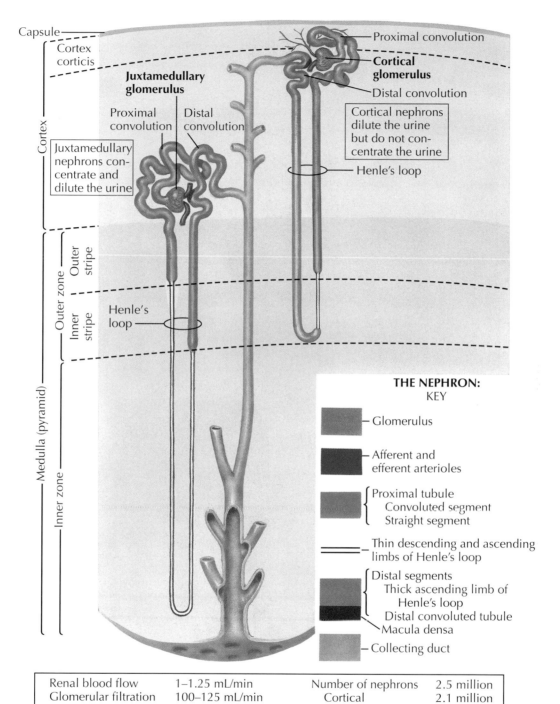

Capsule

Cortex corticis

Cortex

Juxtamedullary glomerulus

Proximal convolution

Distal convolution

Juxtamedullary nephrons concentrate and dilute the urine

Proximal convolution

Cortical glomerulus

Distal convolution

Cortical nephrons dilute the urine but do not concentrate the urine

Henle's loop

Outer stripe

Outer zone

Inner stripe

Henle's loop

Medulla (pyramid)

Inner zone

THE NEPHRON:
KEY

— Glomerulus

— Afferent and efferent arterioles

{ Proximal tubule
Convoluted segment
Straight segment

— Thin descending and ascending limbs of Henle's loop

{ Distal segments
Thick ascending limb of Henle's loop
Distal convoluted tubule
— Macula densa

— Collecting duct

Renal blood flow	1–1.25 mL/min	Number of nephrons	2.5 million
Glomerular filtration rate	100–125 mL/min 140–180 L/day	Cortical Juxtamedullary	2.1 million 0.4 million
Urine flow rate	0.5–18 L/day		

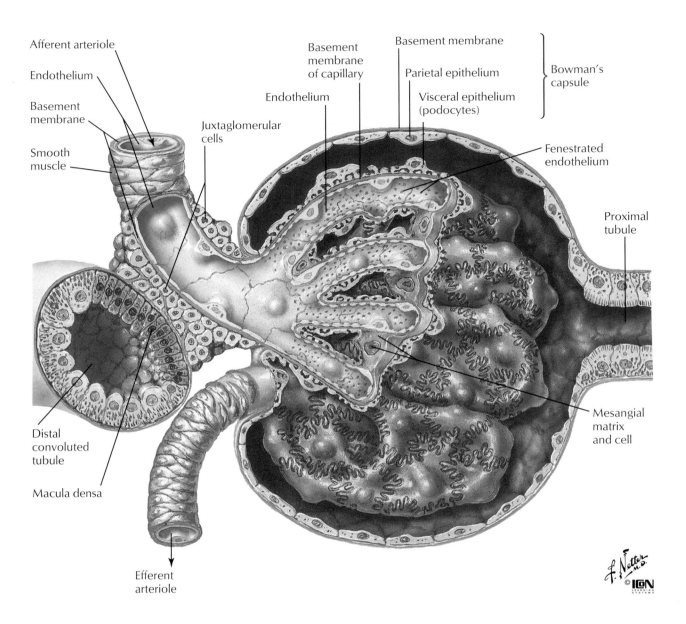

Afferent arteriole

Endothelium

Basement membrane

Smooth muscle

Juxtaglomerular cells

Basement membrane of capillary

Endothelium

Basement membrane

Parietal epithelium

Visceral epithelium (podocytes)

Bowman's capsule

Fenestrated endothelium

Proximal tubule

Mesangial matrix and cell

Distal convoluted tubule

Macula densa

Efferent arteriole

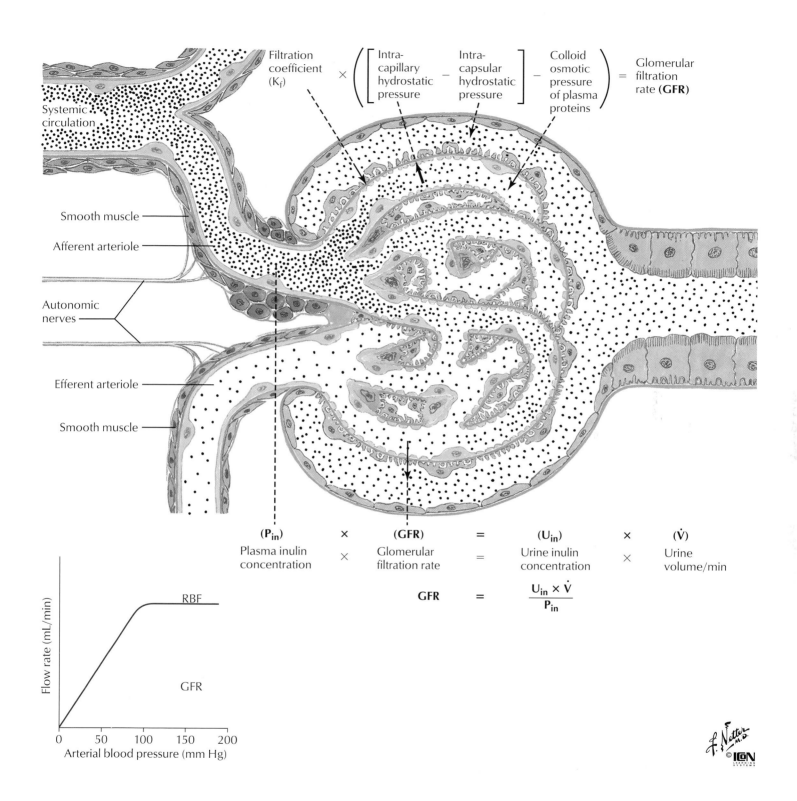

Filtration coefficient (K_f) $\times$ $\left[\begin{array}{c}\text{Intra-}\\\text{capillary}\\\text{hydrostatic}\\\text{pressure}\end{array} - \begin{array}{c}\text{Intra-}\\\text{capsular}\\\text{hydrostatic}\\\text{pressure}\end{array}\right]$ $-$ $\begin{array}{c}\text{Colloid}\\\text{osmotic}\\\text{pressure}\\\text{of plasma}\\\text{proteins}\end{array}$ $=$ Glomerular filtration rate (**GFR**)

Systemic circulation

Smooth muscle

Afferent arteriole

Autonomic nerves

Efferent arteriole

Smooth muscle

(P_{in})	$\times$	(GFR)	$=$	(U_{in})	$\times$	$(\dot{V})$
Plasma inulin concentration	$\times$	Glomerular filtration rate	$=$	Urine inulin concentration	$\times$	Urine volume/min

$$GFR = \frac{U_{in} \times \dot{V}}{P_{in}}$$

RBF

GFR

Flow rate (mL/min)

0   50   100   150   200
Arterial blood pressure (mm Hg)

F. Netter M.D.
© ICON LEARNING SYSTEMS

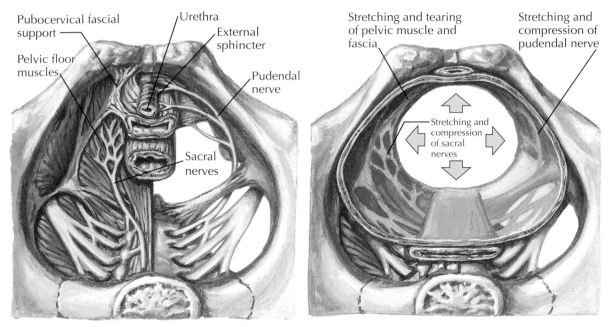

Pubocervical fascial support

Urethra

External sphincter

Pelvic floor muscles

Pudendal nerve

Sacral nerves

Stretching and tearing of pelvic muscle and fascia

Stretching and compression of pudendal nerve

Stretching and compression of sacral nerves

Endopelvic fascia and muscles and nerve supply to internal and external sphincters are susceptible to damage from stretching and compression during delivery

Frontal section of pelvis

Nonpregnant

Pregnant (at delivery)

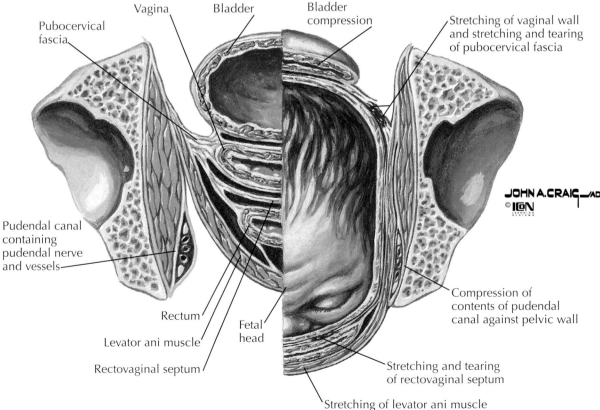

Pubocervical fascia

Vagina

Bladder

Bladder compression

Stretching of vaginal wall and stretching and tearing of pubocervical fascia

Pudendal canal containing pudendal nerve and vessels

Rectum

Levator ani muscle

Rectovaginal septum

Fetal head

Compression of contents of pudendal canal against pelvic wall

Stretching and tearing of rectovaginal septum

Stretching of levator ani muscle

JOHN A. CRAIG—AD
©ICON
LEARNING SYSTEMS

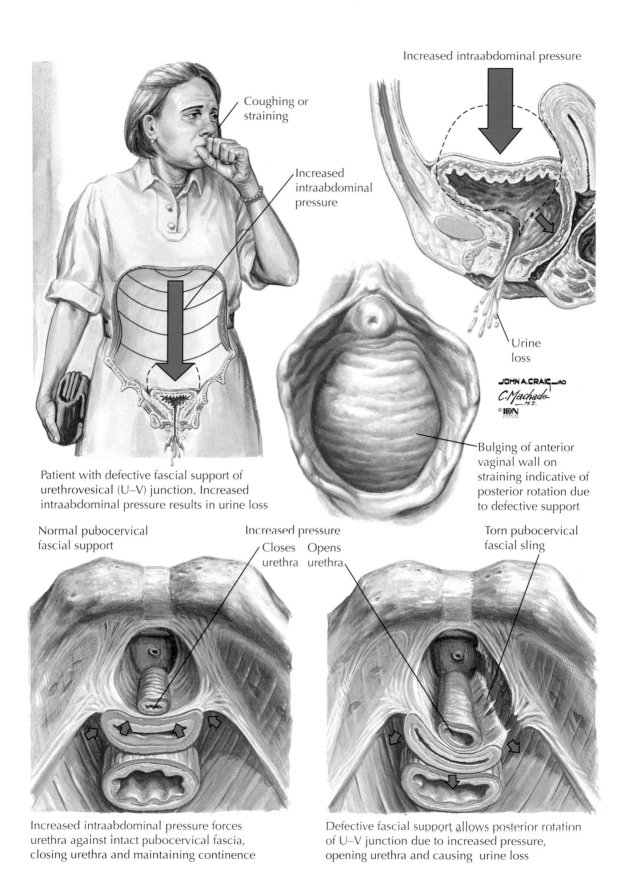

Coughing or straining

Increased intraabdominal pressure

Increased intraabdominal pressure

Urine loss

JOHN A. CRAIG—AD
C. Machado—M.D.
© ICN

Patient with defective fascial support of urethrovesical (U–V) junction. Increased intraabdominal pressure results in urine loss

Bulging of anterior vaginal wall on straining indicative of posterior rotation due to defective support

Normal pubocervical fascial support

Increased pressure
Closes urethra   Opens urethra

Torn pubocervical fascial sling

Increased intraabdominal pressure forces urethra against intact pubocervical fascia, closing urethra and maintaining continence

Defective fascial support allows posterior rotation of U–V junction due to increased pressure, opening urethra and causing urine loss

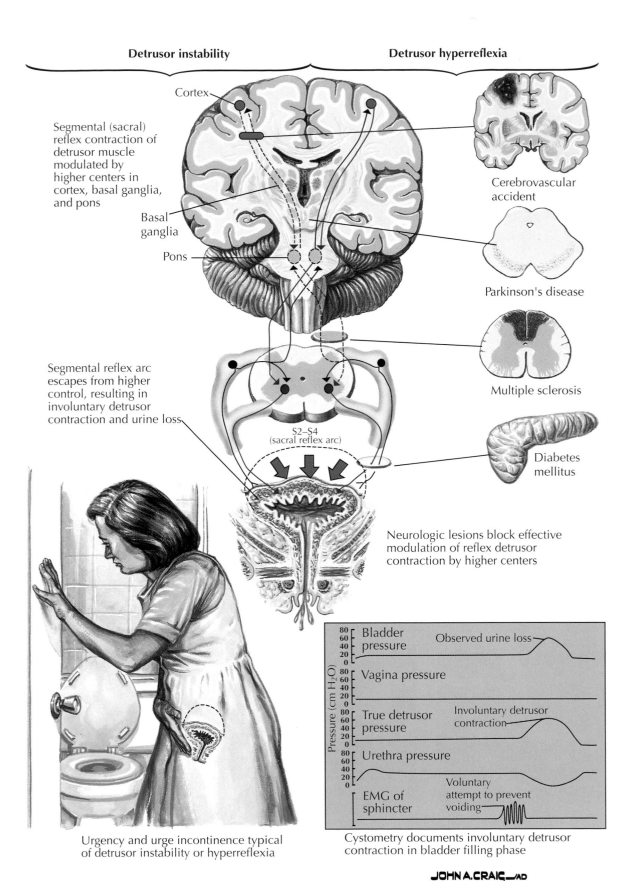

Detrusor instability

Detrusor hyperreflexia

Cortex

Segmental (sacral) reflex contraction of detrusor muscle modulated by higher centers in cortex, basal ganglia, and pons

Basal ganglia

Pons

Cerebrovascular accident

Parkinson's disease

Multiple sclerosis

Diabetes mellitus

Segmental reflex arc escapes from higher control, resulting in involuntary detrusor contraction and urine loss

S2–S4 (sacral reflex arc)

Neurologic lesions block effective modulation of reflex detrusor contraction by higher centers

Urgency and urge incontinence typical of detrusor instability or hyperreflexia

Bladder pressure — Observed urine loss

Vagina pressure

True detrusor pressure — Involuntary detrusor contraction

Urethra pressure

Pressure (cm H₂O)

EMG of sphincter — Voluntary attempt to prevent voiding

Cystometry documents involuntary detrusor contraction in bladder filling phase

JOHN A. CRAIG—AD

C. Machado—M.D.

©ICON

Secondary detrusor instability

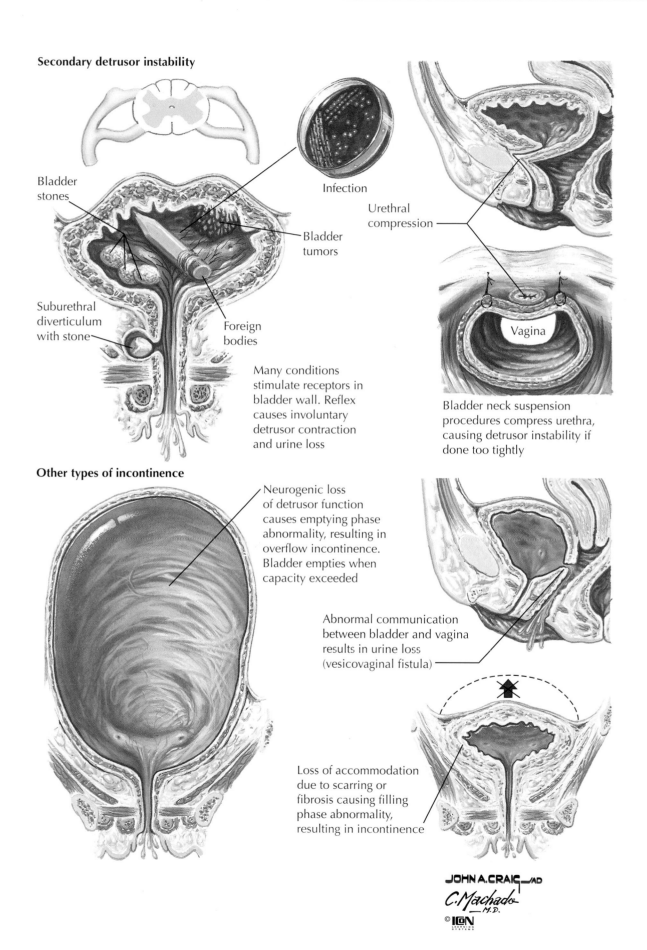

Bladder stones

Infection

Urethral compression

Bladder tumors

Suburethral diverticulum with stone

Foreign bodies

Vagina

Many conditions stimulate receptors in bladder wall. Reflex causes involuntary detrusor contraction and urine loss

Bladder neck suspension procedures compress urethra, causing detrusor instability if done too tightly

Other types of incontinence

Neurogenic loss of detrusor function causes emptying phase abnormality, resulting in overflow incontinence. Bladder empties when capacity exceeded

Abnormal communication between bladder and vagina results in urine loss (vesicovaginal fistula)

Loss of accommodation due to scarring or fibrosis causing filling phase abnormality, resulting in incontinence

JOHN A. CRAIG—MD

C. Machado—M.D.

© ICN

Neurologic evaluation

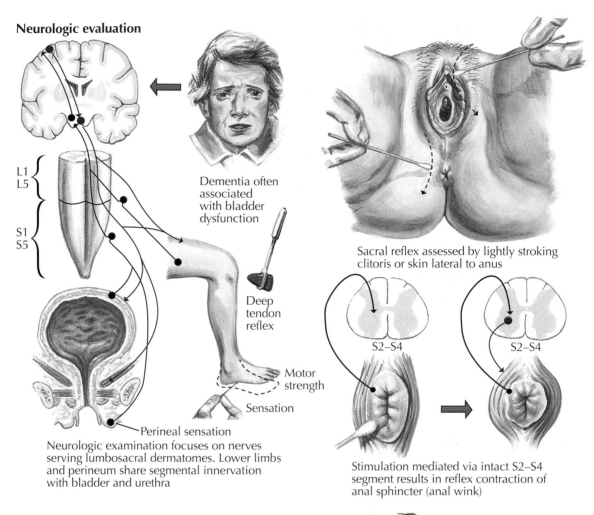

Dementia often associated with bladder dysfunction

Deep tendon reflex

Motor strength

Sensation

Perineal sensation

Neurologic examination focuses on nerves serving lumbosacral dermatomes. Lower limbs and perineum share segmental innervation with bladder and urethra

Sacral reflex assessed by lightly stroking clitoris or skin lateral to anus

S2–S4

S2–S4

Stimulation mediated via intact S2–S4 segment results in reflex contraction of anal sphincter (anal wink)

Abdominal wall examination

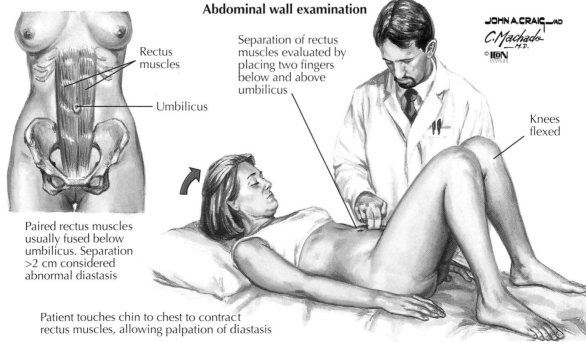

Rectus muscles

Umbilicus

Separation of rectus muscles evaluated by placing two fingers below and above umbilicus

Knees flexed

JOHN A. CRAIG—MD
C. Machado
M.D.
©ICON

Paired rectus muscles usually fused below umbilicus. Separation >2 cm considered abnormal diastasis

Patient touches chin to chest to contract rectus muscles, allowing palpation of diastasis

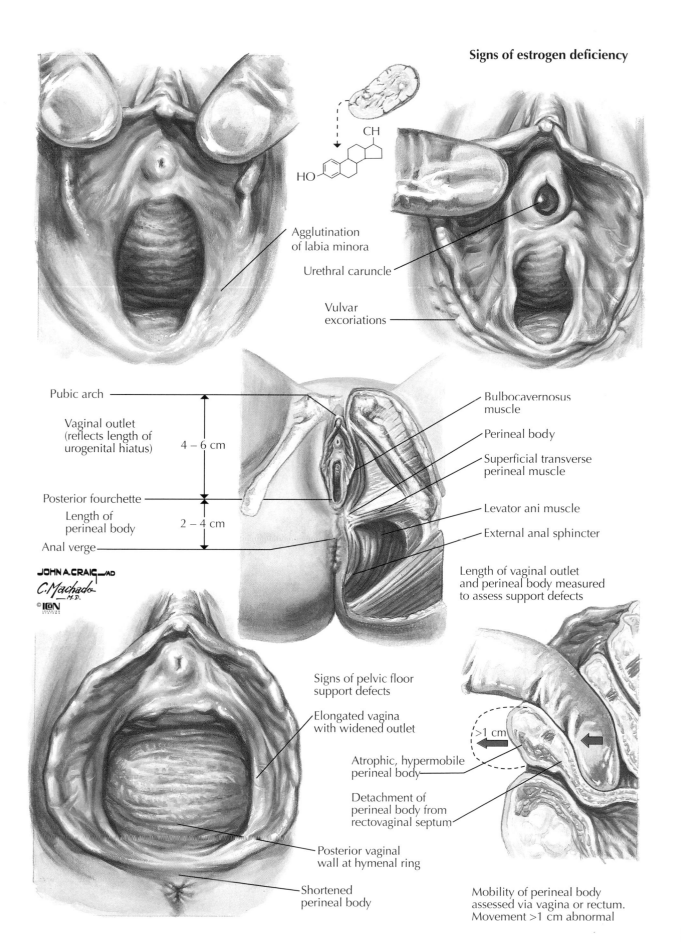

Signs of estrogen deficiency

CH

HO

Agglutination
of labia minora

Urethral caruncle

Vulvar
excoriations

Pubic arch

Vaginal outlet
(reflects length of
urogenital hiatus)

4 – 6 cm

Bulbocavernosus
muscle

Perineal body

Superficial transverse
perineal muscle

Posterior fourchette

Length of
perineal body

2 – 4 cm

Levator ani muscle

External anal sphincter

Anal verge

Length of vaginal outlet
and perineal body measured
to assess support defects

JOHN A. CRAIG—MD
C. Machado
—M.D.
© ICN

Signs of pelvic floor
support defects

Elongated vagina
with widened outlet

>1 cm

Atrophic, hypermobile
perineal body

Detachment of
perineal body from
rectovaginal septum

Posterior vaginal
wall at hymenal ring

Shortened
perineal body

Mobility of perineal body
assessed via vagina or rectum.
Movement >1 cm abnormal

Vaginal length

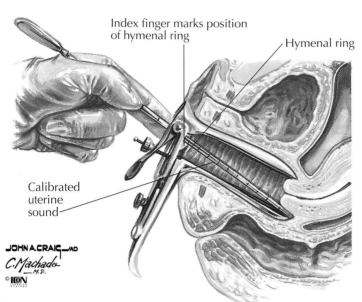

Index finger marks position of hymenal ring

Hymenal ring

Calibrated uterine sound

JOHN A. CRAIG—MD
C. Machado—M.D.
© ICON

With patient at rest, vaginal length from hymenal ring to posterior vaginal fornix measured with uterine sound

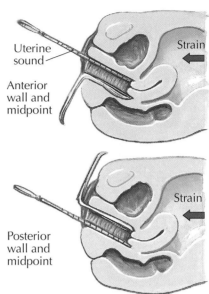

Uterine sound

Anterior wall and midpoint

Strain

Posterior wall and midpoint

Strain

With patient straining, length of anterior and posterior vaginal walls and cervix measured

U–V junction mobility

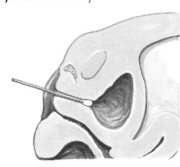

Cotton swab in urethra almost horizontal at rest

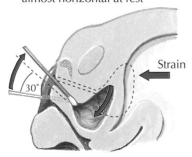

30°

Strain

With cough or Valsalva, swab moves 30° or less. Greater movement indicates U–V junction hypermobility

Lateral defect

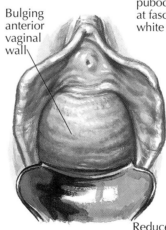

Bulging anterior vaginal wall

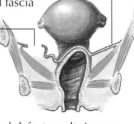

Disruption of pubocervical fascia at fascial white line

Intact fascia

Lateral defect results in poor support of anterior vaginal wall and U-V junction

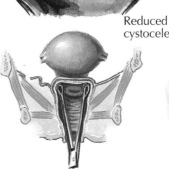

Reduced cystocele

Ring forceps placed in lateral vaginal sulci reapproximates pubocervical fascia to fascial white line and reduces cystocele due to lateral defect

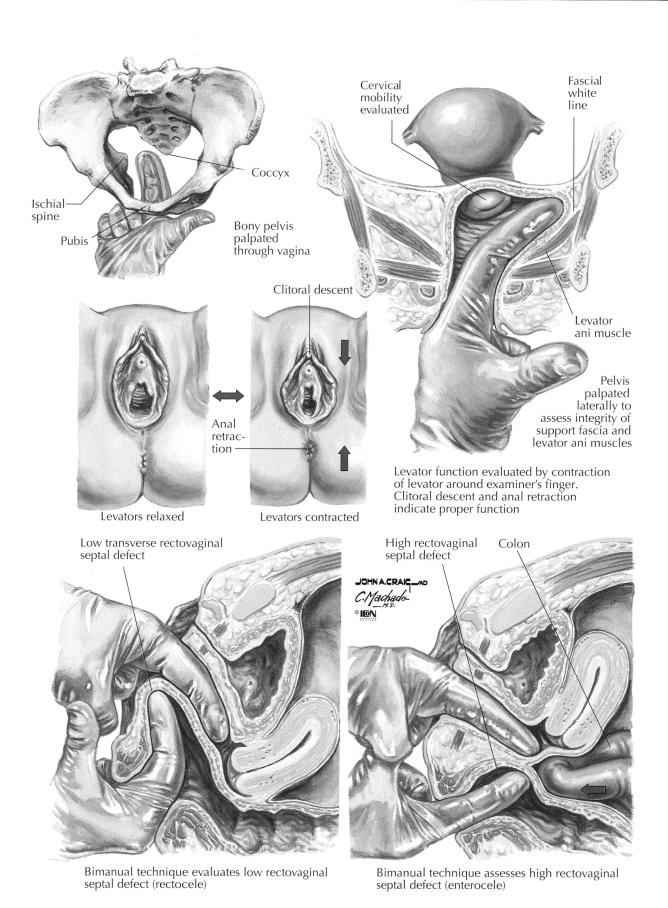

Ischial spine

Pubis

Coccyx

Bony pelvis palpated through vagina

Cervical mobility evaluated

Fascial white line

Levator ani muscle

Pelvis palpated laterally to assess integrity of support fascia and levator ani muscles

Clitoral descent

Anal retraction

Levators relaxed

Levators contracted

Levator function evaluated by contraction of levator around examiner's finger. Clitoral descent and anal retraction indicate proper function

Low transverse rectovaginal septal defect

High rectovaginal septal defect

Colon

JOHN A. CRAIG—MD
C. Machado—M.D.
© ICN

Bimanual technique evaluates low rectovaginal septal defect (rectocele)

Bimanual technique assesses high rectovaginal septal defect (enterocele)

Standing stress test

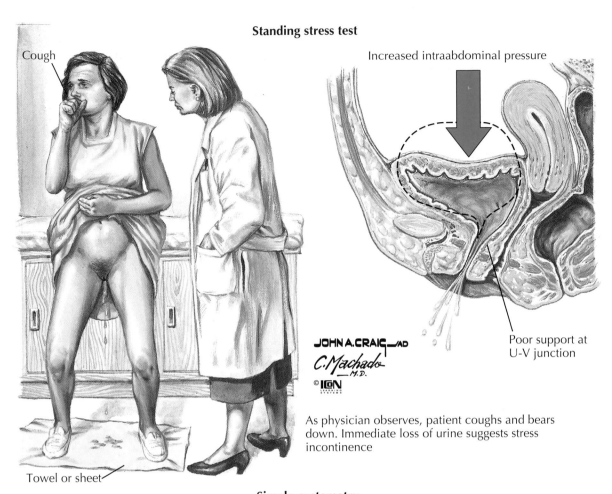

Cough

Increased intraabdominal pressure

Poor support at U-V junction

JOHN A. CRAIG — MD
C. Machado — M.D.
© ICON LEARNING SYSTEMS

As physician observes, patient coughs and bears down. Immediate loss of urine suggests stress incontinence

Towel or sheet

Simple cystometry

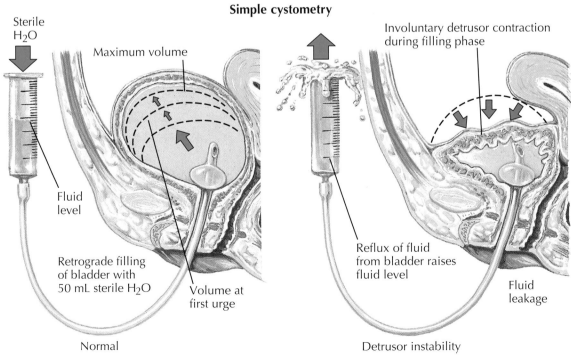

Sterile H₂O

Maximum volume

Fluid level

Retrograde filling of bladder with 50 mL sterile H₂O

Volume at first urge

Normal

Involuntary detrusor contraction during filling phase

Reflux of fluid from bladder raises fluid level

Fluid leakage

Detrusor instability

Pressure readings

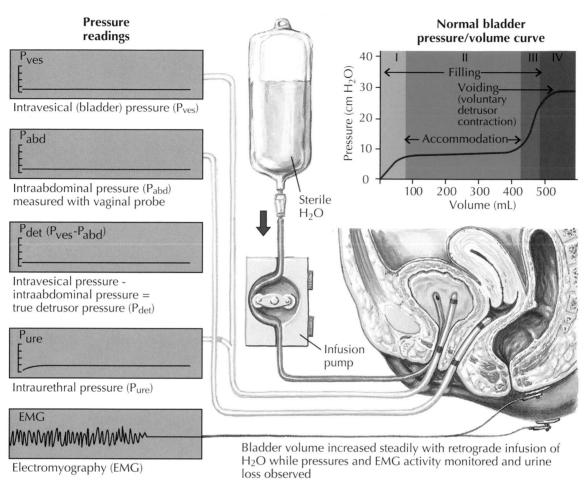

Normal bladder pressure/volume curve

P_{ves}

Intravesical (bladder) pressure (P_{ves})

P_{abd}

Intraabdominal pressure (P_{abd}) measured with vaginal probe

P_{det} (P_{ves}-P_{abd})

Intravesical pressure - intraabdominal pressure = true detrusor pressure (P_{det})

P_{ure}

Intraurethral pressure (P_{ure})

EMG

Electromyography (EMG)

Sterile H_2O

Infusion pump

Bladder volume increased steadily with retrograde infusion of H_2O while pressures and EMG activity monitored and urine loss observed

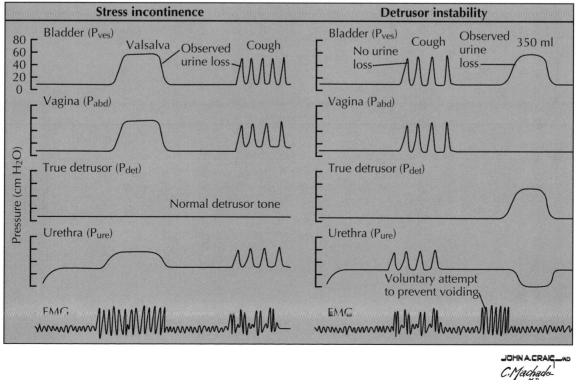

Stress incontinence | Detrusor instability

Bladder (P_{ves}) — Valsalva, Observed urine loss, Cough

Bladder (P_{ves}) — No urine loss, Cough, Observed urine loss, 350 ml

Vagina (P_{abd})

Vagina (P_{abd})

True detrusor (P_{det}) — Normal detrusor tone

True detrusor (P_{det})

Urethra (P_{ure})

Urethra (P_{ure}) — Voluntary attempt to prevent voiding

EMG

EMG

JOHN A. CRAIG__AD
C. Machado M.D.
© ICN

Bladder Drill

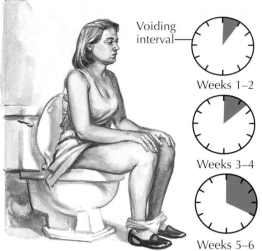

Voiding interval

Weeks 1–2

Weeks 3–4

Weeks 5–6

Voiding by clock rather than urge. Voiding intervals increased gradually based on success with prior interval.

Pelvic Floor Exercises

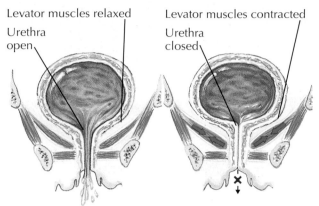

Levator muscles relaxed
Urethra open

Levator muscles contracted
Urethra closed

Patients taught techniques to strengthen levator muscle contraction. Sets of long and short contractions done 2–3 times/day.

Biofeedback Techniques and Other Devices

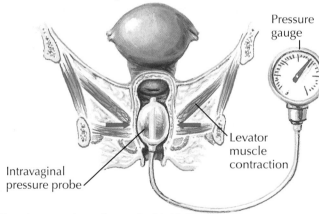

Pressure gauge

Levator muscle contraction

Intravaginal pressure probe

Exercises may be enhanced with biofeedback devices such as vaginal pressure probe to confirm levator muscle contraction

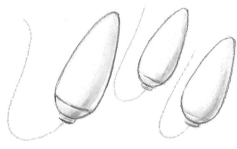

Vaginal cones used to increase levator muscle strength progressively

Pharmacologic Therapy

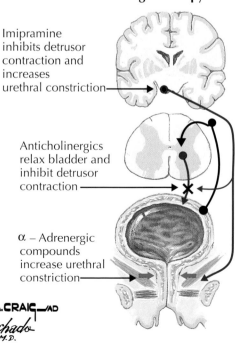

Imipramine inhibits detrusor contraction and increases urethral constriction

Anticholinergics relax bladder and inhibit detrusor contraction

α – Adrenergic compounds increase urethral constriction

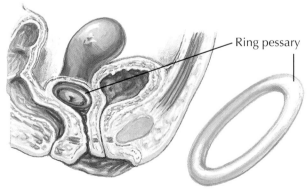

Ring pessary

Pessaries used to reduce prolapse and support pelvic floor muscles

JOHN A. CRAIG — AD
C. Machado — M.D.
© ICON LEARNING SYSTEMS

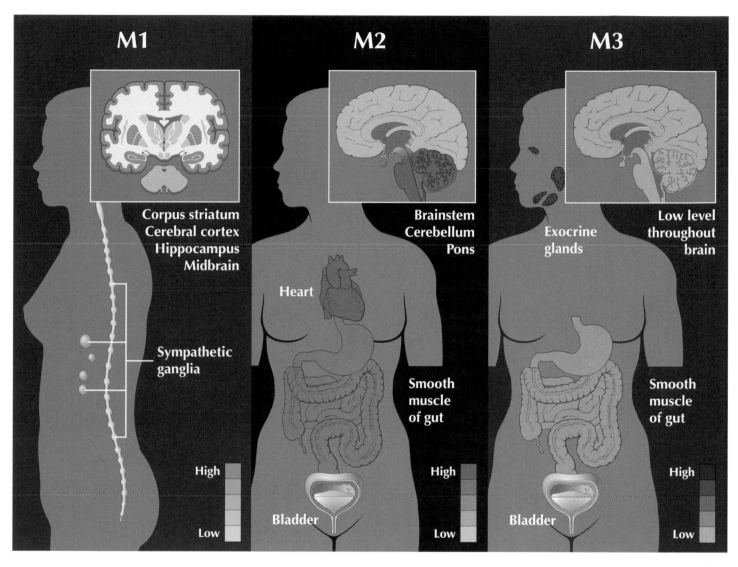

J. Perkins
MS, MFA
© ICN
LEARNING
SYSTEMS

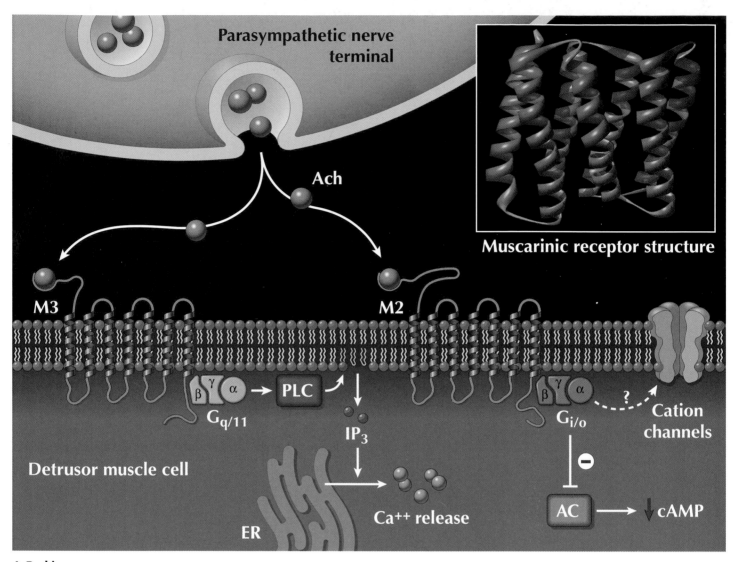

Muscarinic receptor structure

J. Perkins
MS, MFA

© ICN
LEARNING
SYSTEMS